Index

Chapter 1: Introduction to Mindful Eating

Mindful eating, a practice that can revolutionize your relationship with food, is more than just a theoretical concept. It's a practical approach that hones in on your sensory awareness and experience with eating. It's about savoring each bite, being fully present in the moment, and appreciating the nourishment. This practicality of mindful eating makes it a lifestyle change, not just a temporary fix. Adopting mindful eating can enhance your overall wellness and support sustainable weight loss, a gradual, long-term approach to weight management that focuses on healthy eating habits and lifestyle changes rather than quick fixes or restrictive diets. Let's delve into this transformative practice.

The Essence of Mindful Eating

Mindful eating isn't just a diet or a fleeting trend—it is a unique philosophy that intertwines the concepts of mindfulness with the act of eating. Mindfulness involves paying full attention to your present experience without judgment and with a sense of kindness to oneself. When applied to eating, mindfulness helps to recognize and cope with the emotional and physical responses to food. The primary goal of mindful eating is not just to eat less or lose weight but to build healthy eating habits that last a lifetime. It's important to note that mindful eating differs from other eating practices, such as intuitive eating or dieting, focusing on savoring each bite and being fully present in the eating experience.

Historical Roots

The concept of mindful eating has a rich history, rooted in Buddhist teachings that emphasize the importance of mindfulness. The practice is linked to mindfulness meditation, a technique designed to cultivate a heightened awareness of the present moment. Historically, monks practiced eating in silence and focused entirely on the experience, from the taste and texture of the food to the act of chewing and swallowing. Modern psychology and nutrition now embrace this ancient wisdom as a practical approach to managing eating behaviors.

Understanding Hunger

One of the most empowering aspects of mindful eating is gaining a deep understanding of the different types of hunger.

- **Physical Hunger**: Physical hunger, a biological impulse that signals the need for nutrients, builds gradually and is accompanied by clear physical cues like a growling stomach or low energy levels.

Recognizing these signs ensures you adequately nourish your body.

- **Emotional Hunger**: Conversely, emotional hunger stems from emotional needs such as loneliness, boredom, stress, or even happiness. Unlike physical hunger, it feels urgent and demands instant satisfaction. Emotional hunger can lead to mindless eating, where you continue to eat even when full, often driven by cravings for specific comfort foods like sweets or salty snacks. By being aware of these emotional hunger triggers, you can better manage your eating habits and practice mindful eating effectively.

Mindful eating equips you with the tools to recognize and respond to these signals appropriately, giving you the power to choose how you nourish yourself. This understanding of physical and emotional hunger empowers you to make informed decisions about your eating habits, fostering a sense of control and confidence in your relationship with food.

Benefits of Mindful Eating

The benefits of mindful eating are profound. By eating mindfully, people often experience a greater sense of control over their eating habits. It helps identify personal triggers for mindless eating, such as emotions or social pressures. Additionally, mindful eating encourages a healthier relationship with food, characterized by a deep appreciation for the nourishment it provides. This can lead to:

- **Better Digestion**: Eating slowly and mindfully allows your body to digest food more effectively.

- **Reduced Overeating**: By recognizing satiety signals, you can stop eating when you're full, preventing overeating.

- **Increased Meal Satisfaction**: Savoring each bite enhances the pleasure of eating, making meals more satisfying.

Core Principles

The practice of mindful eating is built on several core principles:

- **Awareness**: Focusing on the present moment and acknowledging bodily cues like hunger and fullness.

- **Non-judgment**: Accepting whatever feelings arise without judgment or guilt.

- **Connection**: Recognizing the food sources and the effort to prepare each meal.

- **Patience**: Understanding that developing new eating habits takes time and effort.

- **Gratitude**: Appreciating each element of the food and its journey from source to table.

Starting Your Journey

Embarking on the mindful eating journey is a simple yet profound step towards a healthier relationship with food. It starts with a shift in mindset, observing your current eating patterns without criticism, and gently guiding yourself toward a more conscious approach. You can begin with one meal a day or even one snack. The key is gradually integrating mindfulness into every meal until it becomes a natural part of your lifestyle.

A practical example could be to start by eating breakfast mindfully. Focus on each bite's taste, texture, and smell, and gradually extend this practice to other meals. Here are some steps to begin your journey:

1. **Set Intentions**: Before each meal, take a moment to set an intention to eat mindfully.

2. **Create a Calm Environment**: Find a quiet, distraction-free eating space.

3. **Engage Your Senses**: Notice the colors, smells, textures, and flavors of your food.

4. **Chew Thoroughly**: Take your time to chew each bite completely.

5. **Listen to Your Body**: Listen to your body's hunger and fullness cues.

Deepening the Practice

Transitioning to a mindful eating approach requires both understanding and practice. It's about forming a deeper connection with our food—considering where it comes from, acknowledging the effort involved in its production and preparation, and understanding its effects on our bodies. By recognizing the journey food takes to reach our plates, we can foster a greater appreciation and respect for the nourishment it provides.

Savoring Each Bite

To truly practice mindful eating, one must learn to savor each bite. This involves engaging all the senses—smelling the aroma, noticing the colors and textures, and tasting each flavor note. This sensory engagement makes meals more enjoyable and memorable, and it also helps to regulate the amount of food we consume by increasing satisfaction at meals.

**Techniques for Savoring Each
Bite**

- **Pause Between Bites**: Put
  your utensils between bites
  to slow eating.

- **Take Smaller Bites**: Smaller bites help you appreciate
  the flavors and textures
  more.

- **Breathe**: Take a deep breath
  before eating to center yourself and enhance your awareness.

Discover the Power of Mindful Eating in Your Everyday Life

Integrating mindful eating into daily life can start with small, manageable steps such as:

- **Designate a Quiet, Distraction-Free Eating Area**: Create a calm meal environment.

- **Turn Off Electronic Devices**: Eliminate distractions like phones and TVs.

- **Eat with Others**: Share meals with friends or family

who appreciate and support your mindful eating journey.

These practices help solidify mindful eating as a daily habit, making it more than just a technique—it becomes a lifestyle.

Emotional Eating and Mindfulness

A crucial aspect of mindful eating is empowering ourselves to address emotional eating by learning to pause and identify the source of our cravings. Is it hunger, or is it emotion? By recognizing the difference, we can choose responses that nourish us, whether eating if we're genuinely hungry or addressing emotional needs more appropriately. This understanding puts us in control of our eating habits, empowering us to make healthier choices.

Strategies to Manage Emotional Eating

- **Pause and Reflect**: Before eating, ask yourself if you are starving or eating due to emotions.

- **Find Alternatives**: Engage in activities like walking, journaling, or talking to a friend to address emotional needs.

- **Practice Self-Compassion**: Be kind to yourself when emotional eating occurs. Acknowledge it without judgment and move forward.

Conclusion: A Lifelong Journey

Mindful eating is not a destination but a lifelong journey that can lead to lasting change and more profound satisfaction with eating and life itself. Each meal is an opportunity to practice mindfulness. By engaging fully with our eating experiences, we choose to live our lives more fully and healthily. This lifelong commitment to mindful eating is a testament to our dedication to health and well-being.

This introduction to mindful eating is not just a chapter—it's a call to revolutionize your relationship with food and your life. By embracing the practices and principles discussed, you embark on a transformative journey that can lead to lasting change, profound satisfaction with eating, and a healthier, more aware, and more joyful life.

Chapter 2: Listening to the Body: Physical Hunger vs. Emotional Hunger

Chapter 2: Listening to the Body: Physical Hunger vs. Emotional Hunger. This chapter is crucial to your mindful eating journey, as it will help you understand the fundamental difference between physical and emotional hunger. By learning to recognize their cues and respond appropriately, you can take a significant step towards transforming your relationship with food.

Understanding Physical Hunger

Physical hunger is a biological signal indicating that the body requires nutrients. It is part of the body's natural survival mechanism and can usually be identified by several signs:

- **Stomach Growling**: One of the most recognizable signs of physical hunger is the stomach rumbling, which indicates the stomach is empty.

- **Energy Levels**: Experiencing low energy or feeling weak can also suggest that

your body needs food to re-
fuel.

- **Time Since Last Meal**: Typically, physical hunger develops several hours after the previous meal, suggesting that the body has utilized the energy it previously consumed.

Recognizing these signs and responding promptly ensures you adequately nourish your body.

Emotional Hunger

Unlike physical hunger, emotional hunger arises not from a physical need for food but emotional needs. It is often triggered by feelings such as stress, boredom, sadness, or even joy. Characteristics of emotional hunger include:

- **Sudden Onset**: Emotional hunger can appear abruptly and feel urgent.

- **Specific Cravings**: This type of hunger often manifests as craving specific comfort foods like sweets, salty snacks, or other junk foods.

- **Mindless Eating**: Eating in response to emotional hunger often leads to mindless eating, where one may continue to eat even when full.

Strategies to Distinguish Between Physical and Emotional Hunger

Developing the ability to tell the difference between physical and emotional hunger involves mindful practices and techniques:

- **Pause Before Eating**: Taking a moment to assess why

you're eating can help you determine whether your hunger is physical or emotional.

- **Physical Hunger Test**: Asking yourself if you would eat something healthy can help identify if it's true hunger (if you're starving, almost any food should seem appealing).

- **Emotional Awareness**: Knowing your emotional state before reaching for food can help you identify emotional hunger.

Responding to Physical Hunger

When you determine that your hunger is physical, responding mindfully is crucial:

- **Choose Nourishing Foods**: Opt for whole, nutrient-dense foods that provide lasting energy and support overall health.

- **Eat Mindfully**: Pay attention to the eating process,

savor each bite, and stop eating when comfortably full.

- **Regular Meals**: Eating at regular intervals can help prevent physical hunger from becoming so intense that it triggers overeating.

Practical Tips for Nourishing Foods

- **Breakfast**: Start the day with a meal that includes protein, healthy fats, and fiber, such as oatmeal with nuts and fruits.

- **Lunch**: Opt for a colorful salad with vegetables, lean protein like chicken or tofu, and a healthy fat source like avocado or olive oil.

- **Dinner**: Include a portion of lean protein, a serving of whole grains, and plenty of vegetables. Grilled salmon with quinoa and steamed broccoli makes a balanced dinner.

- **Snacks**: Choose nutrient-dense snacks like Greek yogurt with berries, a handful of nuts, or carrot sticks with hummus.

Managing Emotional Hunger

Managing emotional hunger involves dealing with emotions in ways that do not include food:

- **Find Alternative Responses**: Engage in activities that help you cope with emotions, such as walking, journaling, or talking with a friend.

- **Develop Emotional Resilience**: Techniques such as

meditation, deep breathing, or yoga can improve your ability to manage stress and reduce the likelihood of emotional eating.

- **Seek Professional Help**: If emotional eating is frequent and feels out of control, consulting a therapist or counselor can provide strategies to cope more effectively.

Practical Applications and Exercises

To help you apply these strategies, this chapter includes several practical exercises:

- **Hunger Diary**: Record each time you eat, noting whether the hunger was physical or emotional and what foods you chose. This can help identify patterns and triggers.

- **Mindful Eating Exercises**: Practice eating a single meal daily, focusing entirely on the eating experience, from the flavors and textures to your feelings of fullness.

- **Stress Management Techniques**: Regular practice of stress management techniques can be crucial in preventing emotional eating. This might include scheduled mindfulness meditation or breathing exercises, ideally integrated into your daily routine.

Case Studies

This chapter will also feature case studies of individuals who have successfully distinguished between physical and emotional hunger and adjusted their eating habits accordingly. These real-life examples provide practical insights and inspiration, demonstrating the transformative power of mindful eating practices.

- **Emma's Story:** Emma struggled with emotional eating, often turning to food during stressful times. By keeping a hunger diary and practicing mindful eating exercises, she learned to recognize her emotional triggers and found healthier coping methods, such as taking walks and practicing yoga.

- **Michael's Journey**: Michael used to eat mindlessly, driven by emotional hunger. He developed greater emotional awareness and resilience through therapy and mindfulness practices, reducing his reliance on food for comfort.

Conclusion

Understanding and distinguishing between physical and emotional hunger is crucial in mindful eating. By listening to your body and responding appropriately to its signals, you can develop healthier eating patterns, leading to better weight management and a more profound sense of physical and emotional well-being. This chapter provides the tools and insights to embark on this transformative journey.

Chapter 3: The Rhythm of Meals: When and How to Eat

Establishing a consistent rhythm in eating is as vital as our food choices. This chapter explores the profound impact of meal timing and eating routines on physical and emotional health. By implementing regular, mindful eating patterns, individuals can enhance digestion, manage weight, and increase overall energy levels.

Understanding Eating Rhythms

Eating rhythms involve the patterns and timing of meals and snacks throughout the day. Establishing a regular rhythm helps regulate the body's metabolic processes, supports effective digestion, and can influence our overall energy levels and mood.

- **Circadian Rhythms**: Our bodies operate on circadian rhythms that dictate physical, mental, and behavioral changes over 24 hours. Aligning meal times with our body's natural circadian

rhythms is not just a sugge-
stion; it's a key to enhancing
metabolic health, optimizing
nutrient absorption, and improving sleep quality.

- **Impact on Digestion**: Regular eating times support
the digestive system's natural
cycles. Conversely, erratic
eating patterns can disrupt
digestive processes, leading
to bloating, gas, and irregular
bowel movements.

Benefits of Regular Meal Times

Structured meal times can transform your health and eating habits:

- **Improved Metabolism**: Consistent meal intervals are not just about discipline; they are about stabilizing blood sugar levels, managing insulin production, and maintaining energy balance throughout the day. This, in turn, reduces the risk of metabolic diseases such as type 2 diabetes and obesity.

- **Reduced Snacking and Overeating**: Establishing

fixed meal times can mode-
rate hunger levels throu-
ghout the day, minimizing
cravings and the likelihood
of snacking on unhealthy
foods.

- **Enhanced Energy Levels**:
Regularly scheduled meals
can prevent fluctuations in
energy, warding off the midday slump and sustaining vi-
tality from morning until
night.

**How to Establish Healthy Eating
Rhythms**

Embarking on a structured eating schedule is a journey of self-discovery, where you gain a deeper understanding of your body's needs and daily routine. This process empowers you to take control of your health and well-being.

- **Assessing Your Current Patterns**: Document your current eating habits for a week. Note the times you eat, what you eat, and your hunger levels before and after meals to identify patterns or areas for improvement.

- **Creating a Meal Plan**: Design a meal schedule that fits your lifestyle and meets your nutritional needs. This plan should include three balanced meals and one or two snacks evenly throughout the day.

- **Flexibility Within Structure**: While maintaining a consistent schedule is beneficial, it's also necessary to allow for flexibility. Life is unpredictable, and rigid adherence to specific meal times can create unnecessary stress. Be kind to yourself and adjust your plan when needed.

Mindful Eating Practices During Meals

Mindful eating techniques can enrich the quality of your meals and improve your relationship with food:

- **Eating Without Distractions**: Engage fully with your eating experience by turning off electronic devices and eliminating distractions. This practice helps you focus on your food's taste, texture, and enjoyment.

- **Chewing Thoroughly:** Take the time to chew your food correctly. This aids digestion and makes you more aware of your body's satiety signals, preventing overeating.

- **Listening to Hunger and Fullness Cues:** Regularly check in with your body to gauge your hunger and fullness. This practice fosters a deeper connection with your body and helps you recognize when to begin eating and when to stop, leading to a more balanced diet.

Challenges to Maintaining Eating Rhythms

Several factors can disrupt regular meal times, but strategies exist to manage these challenges effectively:

- **Busy Lifestyles**: For those with unpredictable

schedules, meal prepping and packing portable, healthy options can ensure that you still eat nutritious meals on the go.

- **Social Eating**: Balancing social life and mindful eating is crucial. Choose dining options that align with your eating schedule and preferences, and don't be afraid to suggest eating times that fit your routine.

- **Travel and Time Zones**: Adjusting to different time

zones requires flexibility. Try gradually shifting your meal times a few days before travel to align more closely with your destination's time zone, easing the transition.

Practical Tips for Maintaining Eating Rhythms

Here are some practical tips to help you establish and maintain healthy eating rhythms:

- **Plan Ahead**: Prepare meals and snacks in advance, especially during a busy day. This can prevent you from skipping meals or eating unhealthy fast food options.

- **Set Reminders**: Use alarms or reminders on your phone to prompt you to eat at regular intervals.

- **Stay Hydrated**: Drinking water regularly can help regulate your appetite and keep your body functioning optimally.

- **Listen to Your Body**: Pay attention to your body's

signals. If you're not hungry at a scheduled meal, consider having a smaller portion and adjusting your next meal accordingly.

Case Studies

This section will feature detailed case studies of individuals from various backgrounds who have integrated mindful eating rhythms into their lives. These stories will highlight their challenges, strategies, and the health benefits they have experienced.

- **Sarah's Transformation**: Sarah, a busy professional, struggled with irregular eating patterns due to her hectic schedule. By incorporating meal planning and mindful eating practices, she established a consistent eating rhythm that improved her energy levels and digestion.

- **John's Journey**: John, a frequent traveler, faced challenges maintaining a regular eating schedule. He found ways to align his meal times with his body's natural rhythms through gradual adjustments and flexible planning, enhancing his overall well-being.

Conclusion

The rhythm of your meals plays a critical role in your health and well-being. A mindful eating schedule can substantially improve metabolism, energy, and overall health. Through the strategies and insights provided in this chapter, you can begin to harmonize your eating practices with your body's natural rhythms, leading to a healthier and more balanced life. By making mindful eating a consistent part of your routine, you can enjoy lasting benefits and a deeper connection with your body and food.

Chapter 4: Food as Nourishment: Choosing Foods That Nurture Both Body and Mind

This chapter delves into the importance of selecting foods that nourish the body and the mind. It explores how integrating nutritious foods into your diet can enhance physical health, emotional stability, and overall life quality.

Understanding Nutritional Needs

Understanding the body's nutritional needs is fundamental to selecting foods that nurture. This section breaks down the essential nutrients required for optimal health:

- **Macronutrients:** These are nutrients that our bodies need in more significant amounts to provide energy and support bodily functions:

    - **Proteins:** Essential for building and repairing tissues, proteins are found in

foods such as meat,
fish, dairy products,
legumes, and nuts.

- **Carbohydrates:**
  The body's primary
  energy source, car-
  bohydrates, can be
  complex (found in
  whole grains, vegeta-
  bles, and legumes) or
  simple (found in
  fruits and dairy).

- **Fats:** Necessary for
  brain health, energy,
  and cell function,

healthy fats are found in avocados, nuts, seeds, and olive oil.

- **Micronutrients:** These are vitamins and minerals that our bodies need in smaller amounts:

  - o **Vitamins:** Essential for various bodily functions, vitamins are found in various foods. For example, vitamin C is abundant in citrus fruits, while vitamin D can be obtained from fatty fish and fortified dairy products.

o **Minerals:** Minerals like calcium, potassium, and iron are critical for bone health, muscle function, and oxygen transport in the blood. These are found in dairy products, leafy greens, and red meats.

- **Water:** Vital for every cellular process, water helps maintain hydration, supports digestion, and regulates body temperature. Drinking enough water daily is crucial, and it can also come from water-rich foods like fruits and vegetables.

The Psychology of Eating

Eating is not only a physical need but also an emotional experience. This section explores how foods affect our mood and mental health:

- **Mood-Enhancing Foods:**
Certain foods can positively
impact brain function and
mood:

    o **Omega-3 Fatty
    Acids:** Found in fish
    like salmon and wal-
    nuts, these fatty
    acids are known to
    support brain health
    and reduce symp-
    toms of depression.

    o **Antioxidants:** Ber-
    ries, nuts, and green
    leafy vegetables are

rich in antioxidants that help reduce oxidative stress and inflammation, improving overall mental health.

- **Comfort Foods:** Understanding why certain foods are sought after during times of stress and how to choose healthy alternatives that satisfy emotional needs without compromising health:

    o **Healthy Comfort Foods:** Instead of

reaching for sugary snacks, opt for dark chocolate, which can provide a mood boost with less sugar. Alternatively, a warm bowl of oatmeal topped with fruits can offer comfort and nutrition.

Choosing Whole Foods Over Processed Foods

Processed foods are often convenient, but whole foods provide the best nourishment. This part of the chapter will explain the benefits of choosing whole foods:

- **Nutrient Density:** Whole foods are rich in essential nutrients often lost in processing. For example, a whole apple offers fiber, vitamins, and minerals, whereas apple juice lacks fiber and usually contains added sugars.

- **Natural Fiber:** Consuming whole foods like fruits, vegetables, and grains ensures adequate fiber intake, which aids digestion and prolongs feelings of fullness. Fiber helps regulate the body's use of sugars, keeping hunger and blood sugar in check.

- **Fewer Additives:** Whole foods contain fewer sugars, salts, and fats, reducing the risk of chronic diseases. For instance, homemade tomato sauce from fresh tomatoes has less sodium and preservatives than store-bought versions.

Strategies for Incorporating Nutritious Foods into Every Meal

This section provides practical strategies for including healthy foods in your diet:

- **Meal Planning:** Tips for creating balanced meals that include a variety of nutrients:

    - **Breakfast:** Start the day with a meal that includes protein, healthy fats, and fiber. For example, a bowl of oatmeal topped with nuts, seeds, and fresh fruit.

o **Lunch:** Opt for a colorful salad with vegetables, lean protein like chicken or tofu, and a healthy fat source like avocado or olive oil.

o **Dinner:** Include a portion of lean protein, a serving of whole grains, and plenty of vegetables.

Grilled salmon with quinoa and steamed broccoli makes a balanced dinner.

- **Snacks:** Choose nutrient-dense snacks like Greek yogurt with berries, a handful of nuts, or carrot sticks with hummus.

- **Smart Shopping:** Guidance on selecting the freshest and most nutritious options at the grocery store:

- **Shop the Perimeter:** Fresh produce, meats, dairy, and whole grains are usually found around the store's perimeter. Focus your shopping in these areas.

- **Read Labels:** Look for foods with minimal ingredients and avoid those with added sugars, high sodium levels, or artificial additives.

- o **Seasonal and Local:** Choosing seasonal and locally sourced produce can enhance nutrient intake and support local farmers.

- **Cooking Methods:** Discussing how different cooking methods can preserve or deplete nutrient levels in foods:

- **Steaming:** Retains more vitamins and minerals compared to boiling.

- **Grilling and Roasting:** Enhance flavors without the need for excessive fats.

- **Sautéing:** Use healthy oils like olive or coconut for added nutritional benefits.

Mindful Eating and Food Choices

Linking mindful eating practices with food selection enhances the benefits of a nutritious diet:

- **Mindful Shopping:** Being present during grocery shopping can significantly influence the quality of your food choices. Paying attention to the quality and freshness of the produce and opting for whole foods over processed options can lead to a more nutritious diet.

- **Mindful Cooking:** Engaging fully in cooking can increase appreciation for the food's nutritional value. Take time to prepare meals thoughtfully, enjoying the aromas and the act of creating something nourishing.

- **By embracing the practice of mindful eating, you can enjoy the flavors more profoundly and recognize satiety cues, which in turn helps you make balanced food choices. This** practice encourages you to sit down at a table, chew slowly, and savor each bite without distractions, fostering a deeper appreciation for eating and its impact on your well-being.

Addressing Dietary Restrictions and Allergies

Only some have the exact dietary needs. This section emphasizes the importance of understanding your nutritional needs and guides you on managing common dietary restrictions and allergies while maintaining a nutritious diet.

- **Gluten-Free:** For those with celiac disease or gluten sensitivity, opt for naturally gluten-free grains like quinoa, rice, and buckwheat. Incorporate plenty of fruits, vegetables, and lean proteins to ensure a balanced diet.

- **Dairy-Free:** Choose plant-based alternatives like almond, soy, or oat milk. To meet nutritional needs, include other calcium-rich foods such as leafy greens, almonds, and fortified plant-based milk.

- **Vegetarian and Vegan:** Ensure adequate protein intake through legumes, tofu, tempeh, and quinoa. Incorporate a variety of vegetables, fruits, nuts, and seeds to cover all essential nutrients.

- **Diabetes-Friendly:** Focus on low-glycemic foods like whole grains, legumes, and non-starchy vegetables.

Monitor portion sizes and include lean proteins and healthy fats to stabilize blood sugar levels.

Case Studies

Real-life examples of individuals who have successfully transformed their diets to focus on nourishing foods are not just stories; they are living proof of the practical application of the principles discussed in this chapter. These inspiring narratives offer valuable insights into overcoming challenges and making lasting changes, serving as beacons of

hope and motivation for your journey.

- **Sarah's Transformation:**
  Sarah, a busy professional,
  struggled with stress eating
  and relied heavily on processed foods. She lost weight,
  reported improved energy
  levels, and reduced stress by
  integrating mindful eating
  practices and choosing
  whole, nutrient-dense foods.

- **Tom's Journey:** Tom, a
  middle-aged man with type 2
  diabetes, revamped his diet

by focusing on low-glyce-
mic, whole foods. He stabi-
lized his blood sugar levels
and improved his overall
health through meal plan-
ning and mindful eating. Si-
milarly, Sarah, a young wo-
man struggling with emotional eating, found solace in
mindful eating, which hel-
ped her develop a healthier
relationship with food and
manage her emotions more
effectively.

Conclusion

An essential component of a healthy lifestyle is empowering yourself with the knowledge and tools to make informed food choices. These choices can enhance your physical health, emotional well-being, and overall quality of life. This chapter equips you with an understanding of nutritional needs, the psychology of eating, and practical strategies. By embracing these, you can transform your relationship with food and achieve holistic wellness on your terms. The benefits of mindful

eating are theoretical, tangible, and
life-changing.

Chapter 5: The Art of the Pause: Slowing Down to Savor

In our fast-paced world, taking the time to slow down and savor our food can seem like a luxury. However, the practice of slowing down is a cornerstone of mindful eating. This chapter explores how pausing and genuinely enjoying our meals can lead to better digestion, increased satisfaction, and a healthier relationship with food. It also provides a brief history of mindful eating and

its cultural significance, helping rea-
ders understand the relevance and
importance of this practice.

The Importance of Slowing Down

Eating slowly and mindfully allows us to fully engage with eating, enhancing our sensory experience and improving our body's ability to process food. It's like giving your body time to understand and use your food entirely. Here are some key benefits:

- **Improved Digestion:** When we eat slowly, our

digestive system has more time to break down food, leading to better nutrient absorption and reduced digestive discomfort. This can also help prevent acid reflux and bloating, promoting overall digestive health.

- **Increased Satiety**: Taking time to savor each bite allows our brain to catch up with our stomach, helping us recognize when we're full and preventing overeating.

- **Enhanced Enjoyment**: Eating slowly enhances the flavors and textures of food, making meals more enjoyable and satisfying.

Techniques to Slow Down

Implementing the art of pausing your eating habits requires conscious effort and practice. Here are some techniques to help you slow down and savor your meals:

1. Set a Comfortable Pace

Start by setting a comfortable pace for your meals. Allocate at least 20-

30 minutes to each meal to ensure you have enough time to eat without rushing. This allows your body to process the food better and gives you time to enjoy each bite.

2. Chew Thoroughly

Chewing your food thoroughly is essential for proper digestion. Aim to chew each bite at least 20-30 times before swallowing. This not only aids in breaking down the food but also enhances the flavors and textures, making the meal more enjoyable.

3. Put Down Your Utensils

Between bites, put down your utensils and take a moment to breathe. This simple act can help you slow down and become more aware of your eating pace. It also gives you time to savor each bite and listen to your body's hunger and fullness cues.

4. Take Mindful Breaths

Incorporate mindful breathing into your mealtime routine. Take a deep breath before each bite to center yourself and focus on the present moment. This practice can help you stay mindful and aware throughout the meal.

Creating a Mindful Eating Environment

The environment in which we eat can significantly impact our ability to slow down and savor our food. Creating a mindful eating environment involves minimizing distractions and fostering a sense of calm and presence.

1. Eliminate Distractions

Turn off electronic devices like TVs, phones, and computers during meals. This helps you focus solely on the eating experience and reduces the likelihood of mindless eating.

2. Set the Scene

Create a pleasant and inviting atmosphere for your meals. Set the table with care, use attractive dishware, and consider adding elements like soft lighting or calming music to enhance the dining experience.

3. Eat in Silence

Even for a few minutes, eating in silence can heighten your awareness of the food's flavors, textures, and sensations. This practice can deepen your connection to the meal and increase your enjoyment.

Mindful Eating Practices

Integrating mindful eating practices into your daily routine can help you slow down and savor your food. Here are some exercises to try:

1. The Raisin Exercise

The raisin exercise is a classic mindfulness practice that involves eating a single raisin with full awareness. Start by holding the raisin and observing its appearance, texture, and smell. Then, please place it in your mouth and chew it slowly, paying attention to the flavors and sensations. This exercise can help you cultivate mindfulness and appreciation for your food.

2. Mindful Eating Journal

Keeping a mindful eating journal can help you track your eating habits and reflect on your experiences. Record what you eat, how long it takes, and how you feel before, during, and after the meal. This practice can increase your awareness of eating patterns and help you make mindful choices.

3. Gratitude Practice

Expressing gratitude for your food can enhance your eating experience and deepen your appreciation for the nourishment it provides. Take a moment before each meal to acknowledge the effort that went into producing, preparing, and serving the food. This practice can foster a sense of connection and respect for your food.

Overcoming Challenges

Slowing down and savoring your food can be challenging, especially in a fast-paced world. Here are some common obstacles and strategies to overcome them:

1. Time Constraints

Many people struggle to find time for mindful eating due to busy schedules. To overcome this, prioritize at least one meal a day to eat mindfully. Start with breakfast or dinner, and gradually incorporate mindful eating into other meals.

2. Social Settings

Eating mindfully in social settings can be challenging, as conversations and distractions can interfere with the practice. In these situations, focus on being present and engaged with your companions. Take small pauses during the meal to check in with your body and savor the food.

3. Stress and Emotions

Stress and emotions can trigger mindless eating and make it difficult to slow down. Develop stress management techniques, such as deep breathing, meditation, or physical activity, to healthily cope with stress and emotions. Practice mindful eating even during stressful times to maintain your connection with food.

Conclusion

The art of the pause is a powerful tool in mindful eating. By slowing down and savoring your food, you can enhance digestion, increase satiety, and enjoy your meals more fully. Incorporating mindful eating practices into your daily routine and creating a mindful eating environment can help you develop a

healthier and more satisfying relationship with food. Embrace the art
of the pause and discover the joy of
eating mindfully.

Chapter 6: Emotional Eating and Food: Managing Cravings and Emotions

Emotional eating is a common challenge that many people face. It involves using food to cope with emotions rather than to satisfy physical hunger. This chapter explores the connection between emotions and eating, offering strategies to manage cravings and develop healthier coping methods.

Understanding Emotional Eating

Emotional eating occurs when food is used to deal with feelings rather than satisfy hunger. This behavior can be triggered by various emotions, including stress, boredom, sadness, and even happiness. Understanding the root causes of emotional eating is the first step in managing it effectively.

1. The Emotional Connection

Emotions and eating are deeply intertwined. Certain foods can trigger the release of feel-good chemicals in the brain, such as dopamine and serotonin, which can temporarily relieve negative emotions. However, this relief is often short-lived, leading to a cycle of emotional eating.

2. Common Triggers

Identifying common triggers for emotional eating can help you become more aware of your patterns. Some common triggers include:

- **Stress:** High-stress levels can lead to cravings for comfort foods high in sugar and fat.

- **Boredom**: Eating can distract from boredom or lack of purpose.

- **Loneliness**: Food can substitute for social connection and emotional support.

- **Fatigue**: People may turn to food for a quick energy boost when tired.

Recognizing Emotional vs. Physical Hunger

Differentiating between emotional and physical hunger is crucial for managing emotional eating. Here are some key differences:

- **Emotional Hunger:**

  o Comes on suddenly and feels urgent.

  o Craves specific comfort foods.

  o Is not satisfied even when complete.

  o Is often accompanied by negative emotions.

- **Physical Hunger:**

o Develops gradually and can wait.

o Open to various food options.

o Stops when you are full.

o Is accompanied by physical cues like a growling stomach or low energy.

Strategies to Manage Emotional Eating

Managing emotional eating involves developing healthy coping mechanisms and building emotional resilience. Here are some strategies to help you manage emotional eating:

1. Identify Your Triggers

Keep a journal to track your eating habits and emotions. Note what you eat, when, and how you feel before, during, and after eating. This can help you identify patterns and triggers for emotional eating.

2. Develop Healthy Coping Mechanisms

Finding alternative ways to cope with emotions can reduce the reliance on food for comfort. Some healthy coping mechanisms include:

- **Physical Activity**: Exercise can boost mood and reduce stress. Activities like walking, yoga, or dancing can be particularly effective.

- **Relaxation Techniques**: Deep breathing, meditation, or progressive muscle relaxation can help manage stress and emotions.

- **Creative Outlets**: Engaging in hobbies like painting, writing, or playing music can provide a positive outlet for emotions.

3. Build Emotional Resilience

Building emotional resilience involves developing the ability to cope with stress and emotions healthily. Here are some tips:

- **Practice Mindfulness**: Mindfulness techniques, such as meditation or mindful breathing, can help you stay present and manage emotions more effectively.

- **Foster Social Connections**: Building solid relationships and seeking support from friends and family can provide emotional support and reduce the need for emotional eating.

- **Self-Compassion**: Be kind to yourself and practice self-compassion. Acknowledge that everyone sometimes experiences emotional eating

and use it as an opportunity
to learn and grow.

Mindful Eating and Emotional Awareness

Integrating mindful eating practices with emotional awareness can help you manage emotional eating. Here are some exercises to try:

1. Mindful Check-Ins

Take a moment before eating to check in with yourself. Ask yourself if you are physically hungry or eating due to emotions. This can help you make more conscious choices about when and what to eat.

2. The HALT Method

The HALT method involves asking yourself if you are Hungry, Angry, Lonely, or Tired before eating. This can help you identify if your desire to eat is driven by emotions rather than physical hunger.

3. Mindful Breathing

Practice mindful breathing to center yourself and manage emotions. Take a few deep breaths before eating to calm your mind and focus on the present moment.

Practical Applications and Exercises

Incorporating practical exercises into your routine can help you manage emotional eating effectively. Here are some exercises to try:

1. Emotional Eating Journal

Keep a journal to record your emotions and eating habits. Note the triggers, what you ate, and how you felt before and after eating. This practice can help you identify patterns and develop healthier coping strategies.

2. Mindful Eating Exercises

Practice mindful eating exercises to stay present and aware during meals. Focus on the flavors, textures, and sensations of the food. Pay attention to your body's hunger and fullness cues.

3. Stress Management Techniques

Develop a routine with stress management techniques, such as meditation, deep breathing, or physical activity. Incorporate these practices into your daily life to build emotional resilience and reduce the reliance on food for comfort.

Case Studies

Real-life examples of individuals successfully managing emotional eating can provide inspiration and practical insights. Here are some case studies:

- **Jessica's Story**: Jessica used to turn to food for comfort during stressful times. By keeping an emotional eating journal and practicing mindfulness techniques, she learned to identify her triggers and develop healthier coping mechanisms. Jessica now uses exercise and creative outlets to manage her emotions, reducing her reliance on food.

- **Tom's Journey**: Tom struggled with emotional eating due to loneliness and boredom. He built solid social connections through therapy and mindfulness practices and developed hobbies that provided emotional fulfillment. Tom's journey highlights the importance of emotional resilience and social support in managing emotional eating.

Conclusion

Emotional eating is a common challenge, but it can be managed effectively with the right strategies and practices. You can build a healthier relationship with food by understanding the connection between emotions and eating, recognizing emotional vs. physical hunger, and developing healthy coping mechanisms. Integrating mindful eating practices and emotional awareness can further support your journey toward managing cravings and emotions. Embrace these strategies and discover the path to emotional resilience and a balanced, fulfilling life.

Chapter 7: Mindfulness in Daily Life: Exercises and Routines

Mindful eating is deeply intertwined with mindfulness in daily life. Incorporating mindfulness exercises and routines into your everyday activities can enhance your overall well-being and support your mindful eating practices. This chapter explores mindfulness exercises and routines that can help you stay present, reduce stress, and foster a deeper connection with your food and body.

The Role of Mindfulness in Daily Life

Mindfulness is being fully present and engaged in the current moment. It involves paying attention to your thoughts, feelings, and sensations without judgment. Integrating mindfulness into your daily life can help you manage stress, improve your mental health, and enhance your overall quality of life.

Benefits of Mindfulness

- **Reduced Stress**: Mindfulness practices can help lower

stress levels by promoting relaxation and reducing the production of stress hormones.

- **Improved Mental Health**: Regular mindfulness practice has been shown to reduce symptoms of anxiety and depression, improve mood, and enhance emotional regulation.

- **Enhanced Focus and Concentration**: Mindfulness exercises can improve your concentration and focus at work and in personal activities.

- **Start Your Journey to Better Health: Discover how mindfulness** can lead to healthier lifestyle choices, such as improved eating habits, better sleep, and increased physical activity.

Mindfulness Exercises

Incorporating mindfulness exercises into your daily routine can help you stay present and connected to your

body and mind. Here are some exercises to try:

1. Mindful Breathing

Experience the Power of Mindful Breathing: This simple yet powerful exercise can help you stay grounded and present. Here's how to immerse yourself in the practice:

- **Find a Comfortable Position**: Sit or lie comfortably with your back straight and your hands resting on your lap or sides.

- **Focus on Your Breath**:
  Close your eyes and focus on
  your breath. Notice the sensation of the air entering and
  leaving your nostrils.

- **Breathe Deeply**: Take
  deep, slow breaths, inhaling
  through your nose and exha-
  ling through your mouth.
  Focus on the rhythm of your
  breath and let go of any distractions.

- **Commit to your health
  and wellness journey by
  practicing mindful**

**breathing regularly. Aim
for at least 5-10 minutes
daily, gradually increasing**
the duration as you become
more comfortable with the
practice.

2. Body Scan Meditation

Body scan meditation involves
paying attention to different parts of
your body, promoting relaxation and
body awareness. Here's how to practice it:

- **Find a Quiet Space**: Lie comfortably in a quiet space without being disturbed.

- **Close Your Eyes**: Close your eyes and take a few deep breaths to relax.

- **Focus on Each Body Part**: Start at the top of your head and slowly move your attention down to your toes. Notice any sensations, tension, or discomfort in each area.

- **Release Tension**: As you focus on each body part,

imagine releasing any tension or discomfort. Continue this process until you reach your toes.

- **Practice Regularly**: Incorporate body scan meditation into your daily routine, aiming for at least 10-20 minutes daily.

3. Mindful Walking

Mindful walking is a great way to incorporate mindfulness into your daily routine, especially if you find it challenging to sit still for meditation. Here's how to practice it:

- **Choose a Path**: Find a quiet, safe path to walk without distractions.

- **Focus on Your Steps**: As you walk, bring your attention to the sensation of your feet touching the ground. Notice the movement of your legs and the rhythm of your steps.

- **Engage Your Senses**: Pay attention to the sights,

sounds, and smells around you. Engage all your senses and stay present in the moment.

- **Breathe Deeply**: Take deep breaths as you walk, coordinating your breath with your steps. Inhale for a few steps, then exhale for a few steps.

- **Practice Regularly**: Aim to practice mindful walking for at least 10-15 minutes daily. You can gradually increase the duration as you become more comfortable with the practice.

Mindfulness Routines

In addition to specific exercises, incorporating mindfulness routines into your daily life can help you stay present and connected. Here are some routines to try:

1. Morning Mindfulness Routine

Starting your day with mindfulness can set a positive tone for the rest of the day. Here's a simple morning mindfulness routine:

- **Wake Up Slowly**: Instead of rushing out of bed, take a few moments to stretch and take a few deep breaths.

- **Practice Gratitude**: Consider three things you are grateful for before getting out of bed. This can help shift your mindset to a positive and appreciative state.

- **Mindful Breathing**: Spend 5-10 minutes practicing mindful breathing or meditation to start your day with calm and focus.

- **Mindful Eating**: Have a mindful breakfast, paying attention to the flavors, textures, and sensations of the food. Avoid distractions like TV or smartphones and focus solely on the eating experience.

2. Midday Mindfulness Break

Taking a mindfulness break during the day can help reduce stress and improve your focus. Here's a simple midday mindfulness routine:

- **Find a Quiet Space**: Take a few minutes to find a quiet space to sit comfortably.

- **Practice Mindful Breathing**: Spend 5-10 minutes practicing mindful breathing or a quick body scan meditation to relax and recharge.

- **Mindful Movement**: Incorporate gentle stretches or short walks to release any tension in your body and clear your mind.

3. Evening Mindfulness Routine

Ending your day with mindfulness can help you relax and improve your sleep quality. Here's a simple evening mindfulness routine:

- **Reflect on Your Day**: Spend a few minutes reflecting. Think about what went well, what you are grateful for, and any challenges you faced.

- **Practice Mindful Breathing**: Spend 5-10 minutes practicing mindful breathing or meditation to relax and release any stress or tension from the day.

- **Mindful Reading or Journaling**: Engage in calming activities like reading a book or journaling. Focus on the present moment and let go of any distractions.

- **Mindful Eating**: Have a mindful dinner, paying attention to the flavors, textures, and sensations of the food. Avoid distractions and focus solely on the eating experience.

Incorporating Mindfulness into Daily Activities

Mindfulness can be integrated into various daily activities, helping you stay present and connected throughout the day. Here are some tips for incorporating mindfulness into your daily routine:

1. Mindful Cooking

Cooking can be a meditative and mindful activity. Here's how to practice mindful cooking:

- **Engage Your Senses**: Pay attention to the sights,

sounds, smells, and textures of the ingredients as you prepare your meal.

- **Focus on the Process**: Be present and focused on each step of the cooking process, from chopping vegetables to stirring a pot.

- **Express Gratitude**: Take a moment to appreciate the effort and care that went into preparing the meal and the nourishment it provides.

2. Mindful Cleaning

Cleaning can be a mindful activity that helps you stay present and focused. Here's how to practice mindful cleaning:

- **Set an Intention**: Before you start cleaning, set an intention to be present and mindful throughout the activity.

- **Focus on the Task**: Pay attention to the sensations of cleaning, such as the feel of the cloth, the sound of the vacuum, or the smell of the cleaning products.

- **Breathe Deeply**: Take deep breaths as you clean, coordinating your breath with your movements.

3. Mindful Commuting

Commuting can be a stressful part of the day, but it can also be an opportunity to practice mindfulness. Here's how to practice mindful commuting:

- **Stay Present**: Focus on the present moment and avoid distractions like checking your phone or thinking about your to-do list.

- **Engage Your Senses**: Pay attention to the sights, sounds, and sensations of your commute, whether driving, walking, or taking public transportation.

- **Practice Deep Breathing**: Take deep breaths to stay calm and centered during your commute.

Conclusion

Incorporating mindfulness into your daily life can enhance your overall well-being and support your mindful eating practices. By practicing mindfulness exercises, establishing mindfulness routines, and integrating mindfulness into daily activities, you can stay present, reduce stress, and foster a deeper connection with your food and body. Embrace mindfulness in your daily life and discover the benefits of living mindfully.

Chapter 8: Overcoming Obstacles: Tackling Common Challenges

The journey towards mindful eating and living is rewarding but can also be challenging. This chapter addresses common obstacles people face in maintaining mindfulness and offers practical strategies to overcome them, ensuring you stay on track with your mindful eating practices.

Identifying Common Obstacles

Understanding the common challenges that can hinder your mindfulness journey is the first step in overcoming them. Some of these obstacles include:

- **Busy Lifestyles**: Juggling work, family, and other responsibilities can make finding time for mindfulness practices difficult.

- **Social Pressures**: Social gatherings and peer pressure can lead to overeating or unhealthy food choices.

- **Emotional Stress**: High-stress levels and emotional turmoil can trigger mindless eating and disrupt mindfulness practices.

- **Habitual Patterns**: Long-standing habits and routines can be hard to change, making it challenging to adopt new mindful behaviors.

Strategies to Overcome Busy Lifestyles

A busy lifestyle can make it seem impossible to incorporate mindfulness practices. However, with a few adjustments, you can create space for mindfulness in your daily routine.

1. Prioritize Mindfulness

Make mindfulness a priority by scheduling time for it just as you would for any other important activity. Set aside specific times for mindfulness practices, such as mindful eating, meditation, or exercise.

2. Start Small

Begin with small, manageable changes. Incorporate short mindfulness exercises, such as mindful breathing or a quick body scan, into your daily routine. Gradually increase the duration and frequency of these practices as you become more comfortable.

3. Integrate Mindfulness into Existing Activities

Find ways to incorporate mindfulness into activities you already do. For example, practice mindful breathing while waiting in line or engage in mindful walking during your commute. These small changes can add up and make a significant impact.

4. Set Realistic Goals

Set realistic and achievable goals for your mindfulness practice. Avoid setting high expectations that may lead to frustration or burnout. Instead, focus on gradual progress and celebrate small victories.

Navigating Social Pressures

Social situations can be challenging for maintaining mindful eating practices, especially when surrounded by people who may not share your goals. Here are some strategies to navigate social pressures:

1. Communicate Your Goals

Communicate your mindfulness and healthy eating goals to your friends and family. Explain why these practices are essential to you and how they contribute to your well-being. This can help garner support and understanding from those around you.

2. Plan Ahead

Plan for social gatherings by bringing your healthy dish or eating a small, nutritious meal before attending the event. This can help you make mindful choices and avoid overeating.

3. Practice Portion Control

When faced with abundant food, practice portion control by serving yourself smaller portions and savoring each bite. Focus on the quality of the food rather than the quantity.

4. Mindful Socializing

Engage in mindful socializing by being fully present with your companions. Focus on meaningful conversations and connections rather than solely on the food. This can help shift the emphasis from eating to enjoying the company of others.

Managing Emotional Stress

Emotional stress can significantly trigger mindless eating and disrupt mindfulness practices. Developing healthy coping mechanisms and building emotional resilience can help you manage stress more effectively.

1. Identify Stress Triggers

Identify the sources of your stress and develop strategies to address them. This may involve setting boundaries, delegating tasks, or seeking support from friends, family, or a therapist.

2. Develop Healthy Coping Mechanisms

Find healthy ways to cope with stress, such as physical activity, relaxation techniques, or hobbies. Incorporate these activities into your daily routine to help manage stress and prevent emotional eating.

3. Practice Mindfulness

Incorporate mindfulness practices, such as meditation, deep breathing, or body scan exercises, into your routine to help manage stress and stay present. These practices can promote relaxation and improve your ability to cope with stress.

4. Seek Professional Help

If stress and emotional eating are persistent and difficult to manage, consider seeking professional help. A therapist or counselor can provide guidance and support in developing effective coping strategies and addressing underlying emotional issues.

Breaking Habitual Patterns

Changing long-standing habits and routines can be challenging but is essential for adopting mindful behaviors. Here are some strategies to break habitual patterns:

1. Identify Unhealthy Habits

Identify the habits and routines that are hindering your mindfulness journey. This may include mindless snacking, eating in front of the TV, or skipping meals. Awareness is the first step in making positive changes.

2. Set Clear Intentions

Set clear intentions for the habits you want to change and the new behaviors you want to adopt. Please write down your goals and review them regularly to stay motivated and focused.

3. Create a Supportive Environment

Create an environment that supports your mindfulness goals. This may involve removing unhealthy snacks from your home, setting up a designated space for mindfulness practices, or surrounding yourself with supportive people.

4. Practice Self-Compassion

Be kind to yourself as you work to change your habits. Understand that change takes time and effort, and setbacks are a natural part of the process. Practice self-compassion and use setbacks as opportunities to learn and grow.

Practical Applications and Exercises

Incorporating practical exercises into your routine can help you overcome obstacles and stay on track with your mindfulness journey. Here are some exercises to try:

1. Mindfulness Journal

Keep a mindfulness journal to track your progress, reflect on your experiences, and identify areas for improvement. Record your mindfulness practices, any challenges you encounter, and the strategies you use to overcome them.

2. Mindful Goal Setting

Set mindful goals for your mindfulness practice. Ensure your goals are specific, measurable, achievable, relevant, and time-bound (SMART). Review and adjust your goals regularly to stay motivated and focused.

3. Mindful Visualization

Practice mindful visualization to help you stay motivated and overcome obstacles. Visualize yourself successfully navigating challenges and achieving your mindfulness goals. This practice can boost your confidence and reinforce positive behaviors.

4. Accountability Partner

Find an accountability partner who shares your mindfulness goals. Check-in regularly with each other to discuss your progress, challenges, and strategies for overcoming obstacles. This support can help you stay motivated and committed to your mindfulness journey.

Case Studies

Real-life examples of individuals who have successfully overcome obstacles in their mindfulness journey can provide inspiration and practical insights. Here are some case studies:

- **Amy's Story**: Amy struggled with emotional eating and found it challenging to stay mindful during stressful times. By developing healthy coping mechanisms and practicing mindfulness exercises, she reduced her reliance on food for comfort and built emotional resilience.

- **David's Journey**: David faced social pressures and found it difficult to make mindful choices at social gatherings. By communicating his goals and practicing mindful socializing, he successfully navigated social situations while maintaining his mindfulness practices.

- **Emma's Transformation**: Emma had a busy lifestyle and struggled to find time for mindfulness practices. She created a consistent mindfulness routine that improved her well-being by starting small and integrating mindfulness into her daily activities.

Conclusion

Overcoming obstacles is an essential part of the mindfulness journey. By identifying common challenges and implementing practical strategies, you can stay on track with your mindful eating and living practices. Embrace this chapter's strategies and exercises to navigate busy life-styles, social pressures, emotional stress, and habitual patterns. Remember that setbacks are a natural part of the process, and practice self-compassion as you work towards your mindfulness goals. With dedication and perseverance, you can overcome obstacles and enjoy the lasting benefits of mindful eating and living.

Chapter 9: Success Stories: Real-Life Transformations

Real-life stories of transformation can be a powerful source of inspiration and motivation. This chapter explores various success stories of individuals who have embraced mindful eating and experienced profound life changes. These stories highlight the challenges they faced, the strategies they employed, and the incredible outcomes they achieved.

Emma's Journey to Overcoming Emotional Eating

Emma, a 35-year-old marketing executive, struggled with emotional eating for years. Her demanding job often left her feeling stressed and overwhelmed, leading her to seek comfort in food. Late-night snacking became a habit, and she gained significant weight, affecting her self-esteem and health.

The Turning Point

Emma decided to make a change after a routine health checkup revealed that she was at risk for type 2 diabetes. She realized that her emotional eating habits were not only affecting her weight but also her overall health.

Strategies and Practices

Emma began by keeping a food diary to track her eating habits and identify her emotional triggers. She also started practicing mindful eating techniques:

- **Mindful Breathing**: Before meals, Emma took a few deep breaths to center herself and focus on the present moment.

- **Savoring Each Bite**: She made a conscious effort to slow down, chew thoroughly, and appreciate the flavors and textures of her food.

- **Emotional Awareness**: Emma learned to differentiate between physical and emotional hunger, finding alternative ways to cope with stress, such as yoga and journaling.

The Transformation

Within a few months, Emma noticed significant changes. She lost weight, her energy levels increased, and her risk of diabetes decreased. Most importantly, she developed a healthier relationship with food and learned to manage her emotions without relying on eating.

John's Path to Better Digestion and Health

John, a 50-year-old teacher, had been dealing with digestive issues for years. Frequent bloating, indigestion, and irregular bowel movements were part of his daily life.

Traditional treatments provided only temporary relief, and he sought a more sustainable solution.

The Turning Point

John's interest in holistic health led him to discover mindful eating. He learned that slowing down and paying attention to his eating habits could significantly improve his digestion.

Strategies and Practices

John incorporated several mindful eating practices into his daily routine:

- **Chewing Thoroughly**: He started chewing each bite at least 20 times to aid digestion.

- **Eating Without Distractions**: John created a calm eating environment, free from TV and electronic devices, to focus solely on his meals.

- **Listening to His Body**: He listened to his body's hunger and fullness cues, avoiding overeating and choosing nourishing foods.

168

The Transformation

After a few months, John experienced a remarkable improvement in his digestive health. Bloating and indigestion became rare occurrences, and he enjoyed regular bowel movements. John also felt more energized and discovered a newfound joy in eating mindfully.

Sarah's Success with Weight Management

Sarah, a 28-year-old nurse, had been grappling with weight management since her teenage years. Her journey was not a smooth one, as she had tried various diets with limited success, often finding herself in a cycle of weight loss and gain.

The Turning Point

Frustrated with the yo-yo dieting, Sarah sought a more sustainable approach. She attended a workshop on mindful eating, which sparked her interest in changing her relationship with food.

Strategies and Practices

Sarah adopted several mindful eating strategies to support her weight management goals:

- **Regular Meals**: She established a regular eating schedule, including three balanced meals and healthy snacks.

- **Mindful Portions**: Sarah practiced portion control by slowly serving smaller portions and eating to recognize satiety signals.

- **Gratitude Practice**: Before each meal, she took a moment to express gratitude for her food, fostering a deeper appreciation for the nourishment it provided.

The Transformation

Sarah's unwavering commitment to mindful eating led to a remarkable transformation. Over a year, she shed 30 pounds and maintained her weight without feeling deprived. More than just a physical change, she also experienced a boost in self-esteem and a healthier body image.

Michael's Journey to Managing Stress Through Mindful Eating

Michael, a 42-year-old lawyer, grappled with the intense stress of his demanding job. This stress often manifested in unhealthy eating habits, such as skipping meals or resorting to binge eating, a coping mechanism that only exacerbated his stress levels.

The Turning Point

After experiencing burnout and significant weight gain, Michael prioritized his health. He learned about

mindful eating through a colleague
and decided to try it.

Strategies and Practices

Michael integrated mindful eating
into his stress management routine:

- **Mindful Breathing**: He
  practiced mindful breathing
  exercises before meals to reduce stress and improve focus.

- **Mindful Meals**: Michael al-
  located specific meal times,
  ensuring he ate regularly and

mindfully, even on busy days.

- **Healthy Alternatives**: He replaced stress-induced junk food with healthy snacks like fruits and nuts.

The Transformation

Michael's mindful eating practice significantly reduced his stress levels. He regained control over his eating habits, lost weight, and found a more balanced approach to work and life. His energy and productivity improved, and he felt more at peace with himself.

Conclusion

These success stories illustrate the transformative power of mindful eating. By incorporating mindful eating practices, individuals like Emma, John, Sarah, and Michael have overcome various challenges and achieved remarkable improvements in their health and well-being. These real-life examples inspire and motivate, demonstrating that mindful eating can lead to profound and lasting change.

Chapter 10: Sustaining Change: Long-Term Strategies for Mindful Eating

Adopting mindful eating is a significant step towards better health and well-being, but sustaining these changes long-term requires ongoing commitment and strategies. This chapter focuses on maintaining mindful eating practices over time, ensuring lasting benefits and continued progress.

The Importance of Long-Term Commitment

Sustaining mindful eating practices is not a short-term endeavor; it's a long-term commitment. Here's why it's crucial:

- **Consistent Benefits**: Long-term practice ensures that the benefits of mindful eating, such as improved digestion, better weight management, and emotional well-being, are sustained.

- **Habit Formation**: Repetition and consistency help transform mindful eating from a conscious effort into an automatic habit.

- **Continued Growth**: Ongoing practice allows continuous learning and growth, deepening your relationship with food and yourself.

Establishing a Support System

A support system can significantly enhance your ability to sustain mindful eating practices. Here are some strategies to build and maintain support:

1. Family and Friends

Involve your family and friends in your mindful eating journey. Share your goals and practices with them and encourage them to join you. This can create a supportive environment and foster mutual accountability.

2. Mindful Eating Groups

Join or create a mindful eating group. Regular meetings with like-minded individuals can provide encouragement, share experiences, and offer new insights. Online communities and local workshops can also be valuable resources.

3. Professional Guidance

Consider seeking guidance from nutritionists, therapists, or mindfulness coaches. These individuals have expertise in mindful eating and can provide personalized advice, help you overcome challenges, and motivate you.

Integrating Mindful Eating into Your Routine

Making mindful eating a consistent part of your daily routine is crucial for long-term success. Here are some tips:

1. Meal Planning

Plan your meals ahead of time to ensure they are balanced and nutritious. Meal planning helps you avoid last-minute unhealthy choices and ensures you have the ingredients for mindful meals, promoting a healthier eating habit.

2. Consistent Meal Times

Establish regular meal times to create a structured eating routine. Consistency helps regulate your body's hunger and fullness cues, making it easier to eat mindfully.

3. Mindful Eating Rituals

Develop rituals around your meals to enhance mindfulness. This could include setting the table, expressing gratitude, or taking a few deep breaths before eating. Rituals can make meals more meaningful and help you stay present.

Continuing Education and Practice

Continual learning and practice are essential for maintaining mindful eating. Here are some strategies:

1. Read and Learn

Stay informed by reading books, articles, and research on mindful eating and nutrition. Continuous learning can reinforce your practices and introduce new ideas.

2. Attend Workshops and Classes

Participate in workshops and classes on mindfulness and mindful eating. These can provide fresh perspectives, deepen your understanding, and keep you engaged.

3. Practice Regularly

Regular practice is crucial in sustaining mindful eating. Set aside time each day for mindfulness exercises, such as meditation or mindful breathing, to support your eating practices.

Adapting to Life Changes

Life is dynamic, and circumstances change. Adapting your mindful eating practices to fit new situations is crucial for long-term success.

1. Flexibility

Be flexible with your mindful eating practices. Understand that some days may be more challenging, and adjusting your approach as needed is okay. Flexibility helps you stay committed without feeling overwhelmed.

2. Life Transitions

Major life transitions can disrupt your routine, such as moving, changing jobs, or becoming a parent. Plan and find ways to incorporate mindful eating into your new circumstances. For example, prioritize setting up a space for mindful meals during a move.

3. Continuous Reflection

Regularly reflect on your mindful eating journey. Assess what's working well and what needs adjustment. Reflection helps you stay aware of your progress and areas for improvement.

Overcoming Setbacks

Setbacks are a natural part of any journey. Here's how to overcome them and stay on track:

1. Practice Self-Compassion

When setbacks occur, remember to be kind to yourself. Understand that they are part of the process and an opportunity for growth. Practicing self-compassion is vital to staying resilient and committed to your mindful eating journey.

2. Identify Triggers

Identify the triggers that lead to setbacks in your mindful eating journey. These could include stress from work, social pressures to indulge in unhealthy foods, or emotional challenges that affect your eating habits. Understanding your triggers allows you to develop strategies to manage them effectively.

3. Recommit to Your Goals

After a setback, take time to recommit to your mindful eating goals. Revisit your reasons for adopting mindful eating and reaffirm your commitment to health and wellbeing.

Celebrating Progress

Celebrating your progress is essential for maintaining motivation and a positive mindset. Here's how to celebrate your mindful eating journey:

1. Recognize Achievements

Acknowledge both minor and significant achievements. Celebrate your progress, whether maintaining a regular meal schedule or navigating a challenging social event.

2. Reward Yourself

Reward yourself for your efforts. Choose rewards that support your overall well-being, such as a relaxing day at the spa, a new book, or a healthy cooking class.

3. Share Your Success

Share your successes with your support system. Celebrating with others can reinforce your accomplishments and provide additional motivation.

Conclusion: Embracing Mindful Eating for Life

Sustaining mindful eating practices is a lifelong journey that requires commitment, flexibility, and continual learning. You can maintain your mindful eating habits by building a support system, integrating mindful eating into your routine, adapting to life changes, overcoming setbacks, and celebrating progress. These habits refer to being fully present and aware of your eating experience, including the taste, texture, and smell of food and your body's hunger and fullness cues. Embrace mindful eating as a way of life, and discover its profound impact on your health, well-being, and overall quality of life.